Heart Disease
in Pregnancy

Complications and Management

Akmal El-Mazny

CONTENTS

INTRODUCTION

Pregnancy makes profound changes in the cardiovascular system that have the potential to adversely affect maternal and fetal health, especially in the presence of underlying heart conditions.

Valvular heart disease in pregnancy is relatively infrequent, and tends to have a favorable prognosis if the risks are appropriately managed.

Patients with congenital heart disease were traditionally advised against pregnancy; however, as our understanding of the unique issues facing this population has improved, many of those limitations have been removed.

The presence of cardiovascular disease in pregnant women poses a difficult clinical scenario in which the responsibility of the treating physician extends to the unborn fetus.

Therefore, women with cardiovascular compromise due to cardiac disease need specialist input and careful pre-, peri-, and post-partum follow-up.

I hope that this book will provide a comprehensive review of heart disease in pregnancy along with its complications and management, and that you will be able to apply this information to your professional practice.

THE HEART AND PREGNANCY

CARDIOVASCULAR CHANGES DURING PREGNANCY

Pregnancy has a striking effect on the circulatory system; most of these hemodynamic changes start in the first trimester, peak during the second trimester, and plateau during the third trimester.

Peripheral vasodilation (induced by progesterone) leading to a decrease in systemic vascular resistance is thought to be the first cardiovascular change associated with pregnancy.

Cardiac output increases by 20% at 8 weeks gestation and by up to 40-50% at 20-28 weeks gestation; twin pregnancies result in an additional 15% rise in maternal cardiac output.

This is achieved predominantly via an increase in stroke volume due to an increase in ventricular end-diastolic volume, wall muscle mass, and contractility.

Additionally, heart rate normally increases by 10-15 beats per minute particularly in late pregnancy, and atrial as well as ventricular arrhythmias may increase in frequency in predisposed patients.

During the third trimester, cardiac output is further influenced by body position, where the supine position causes caval compression by the gravid uterus; this leads to a decrease in venous return, which can cause supine hypotension of pregnancy.

Blood pressure decreases by 10-15 mm Hg owing to a decrease in systemic vascular resistance caused by the creation of a low resistance circuit by the placenta and vasodilatation.

Plasma volume increases approximately 40% and red blood cell volume 30% above baseline prepregnancy levels.

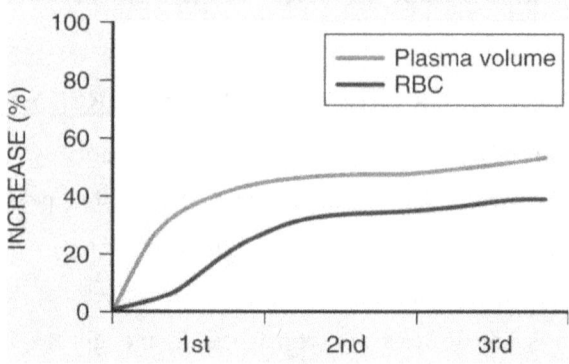

Plasma and RBC volume changes during the three trimesters

This disproportionate increase in plasma volume, that exceeds the rise in red cell mass, results in mild relative anemia and low hematocrit level.

The plasma volume increases to approximately 50% above baseline by the second trimester and then virtually plateaus until delivery.

Estrogen-mediated stimulation of the rennin angiotensin axis results in increased renal tubular absorption of sodium and an increase in total body salt and water, contributing to the increased plasma volume.

Chest radiographic studies reveal a mild increase in cardiac size, a horizontal shift of the heart that increases with the duration of pregnancy, and fullness of the left cardiac border and pulmonary vascular supply.

The delivery and immediate postpartum period is associated with further profound and rapid changes in the circulatory system.

During delivery, cardiac output, heart rate, blood pressure, and systemic vascular resistance increase with each uterine contraction.

Delivery-related pain and anxiety aggravate the increase in heart rate and blood pressure.

Labor leads to further increases in cardiac output by 15% in the first stage and 50% in the second stage.

Immediately postpartum, the delivery of the placenta increases afterload by removing the low resistance circulation and increases the preload by returning placental blood to the maternal circulation may increase cardiac output by as much as 60-80%.

This increase in preload is accentuated by the elimination of the mechanical compression of the inferior vena cava.

After delivery, stroke volume decreases from pregnancy levels to normal levels by 2 weeks postpartum.

Heart rate remains elevated for 2 days postpartum and returns to baseline by 10 days after delivery.

Cardiac output similarly decreases from pregnancy levels to normal levels between 24 hours and 10 days postpartum.

The impact of these physiological changes to a pregnant woman with cardiac disease will vary according to the type and severity of the disease.

These changes can place an intolerable strain on an abnormal heart, necessitating invasive hemodynamic monitoring and aggressive medical management.

CARDIOVASCULAR EVALUATION DURING PREGNANCY

The patient's history is an essential part of the initial risk assessment and should include information on the baseline functional status and previous cardiac events because these are strong predictors of peripartum cardiac events.

The strongest predictors include the following:

- Any prior cardiac event
- Cyanosis or poor functional class
- Left-sided heart obstruction
- Ventricular dysfunction

Left-sided heart obstruction includes valve disease or hypertrophic cardiomyopathy (aortic valve area <1.5 cm^2, mitral valve area <2 cm^2, or left ventricular outflow tract peak gradient >30 mm Hg).

Impaired ventricular function is significant when the ejection fraction is below 40%.

Prior events of interest also include treatment for heart failure, TIA or stroke, or arrhythmia.

The 2011 update to the American Heart Association guideline for the prevention of cardiovascular disease in women recommends that risk assessment at any stage of life include a detailed history of pregnancy complications.

Gestational diabetes, preeclampsia, preterm birth, and birth of an infant small for gestational age are ranked as major risk factors for cardiovascular disease.

Many of the normal symptoms of pregnancy, such as dyspnea on exertion, orthopnea, ankle edema, and palpitations, are also symptoms of cardiac decompensation.

However, angina, resting dyspnea, paroxysmal nocturnal dyspnea, or a sustained arrhythmia are not expected with pregnancy and warrant a further diagnostic workup.

Almost all pregnant women develop physiologic murmurs, which are usually soft, midsystolic murmurs heard along the left sternal border usually caused by functional pulmonary stenosis due to increased transvalvular flow.

Physical signs commonly seen with pregnancy are jugular venous distension, an apical S_3, basal crackles, prominent left and right ventricular apical impulses, exaggerated heart sounds, and peripheral edema.

Diastolic murmurs are rare with pregnancy despite the increased blood flow through the atrioventricular valves; their presence should prompt further diagnostic evaluation.

Systolic murmurs more than 2/6 in intensity, continuous murmurs, and murmurs that are associated with symptoms or electrocardiographic changes should also prompt further investigation such as echocardiography.

Electrocardiography offers low-cost screening that may identify the need for further study if findings otherwise appear benign.

In pregnancy, the axis can shift right or left but usually stays in the normal range.

During normal pregnancy, multiple changes can be seen such as increased R wave amplitude in leads V_1 and V_2, T wave inversion in lead V_2, and a small Q wave and inverted P wave in lead III.

Pregnancy is associated with a higher rate of maternal arrhythmias, ranging from 73-93% in some studies.

If impaired functional status is a concern or the patient's history is unreliable, baseline oxygen saturation and low-level exercise testing with oxygen monitoring and oxygen consumption may be helpful.

Cardiac catheterization should be avoided in pregnancy and should be reserved only for situations in which therapeutic intervention is being considered.

Findings such as ventricular hypertrophy, evidence of a prior myocardial infarction or ischemia, atrial enlargements, conduction abnormalities, or arrhythmias should prompt a more extensive workup.

GENERAL PRINCIPLES OF MANAGEMENT

Pre-delivery

All women of reproductive age with congenital or acquired heart disease should have access to specialized multidisciplinary preconception counselling in order to empower them to make choices about pregnancy.

Once they are pregnant, all women with heart disease should be assessed clinically as soon as possible by a multidisciplinary team and appropriate investigations undertaken.

The core members of the team should include suitably experienced obstetricians, cardiologists, and anaesthetists; but neonatologists, and intensivists should also be involved in planning, when appropriate.

A clear plan for the management of labor and the puerperium in women with heart disease should be established in advance, well documented, and distributed widely (including to the woman herself) so that all personnel likely to be involved in the woman's intra- and post-partum care are fully informed.

The main aims of management are: to optimize the mother's condition during the pregnancy (e.g. considering ß-blockers, thromboprophylaxis, or pulmonary arterial vasodilators in appropriate cases); to monitor for deterioration; and minimize any additional load on the cardiovascular system from delivery and the post-partum period.

Women with heart failure can be safely treated with diuretics, digoxin, and hydralazine, nitrates, or both as vasodilators to offload the left ventricle.

Additional fetal assessments may be needed in order to monitor for potential problems arising from pharmacological treatment of the mother.

Potential Fetal Effects of Cardiovascular Drugs during Pregnancy

Cardiovascular Drugs	Fetal Effects
ACE-inhibitors	– Avoid in all trimesters if possible – Skull defects, oligohydramnios – May adversely affect fetal and neonatal arterial pressure control and renal function
Warfarin	– Teratogenic in first trimester – Risk of fetal haemorrhage – Increased risk miscarriage and stillbirth
ß-blockers	– May cause intra-uterine growth restriction, neonatal hypoglycaemia, and bradycardia
Sildenafil	– Toxicity in animal studies – No reports of toxicity in humans
Diuretics	– Thiazides in the third trimester may cause neonatal thrombocytopenia
Digoxin	– No reports of harm to fetus – May need dosage adjustment
Hydralazine	– No reports of serious harm in third trimester – Manufacturer advises avoid in first and second
LMWH	– Not known to be harmful to fetus
Unfractionated heparin	– Not known to be harmful to fetus
Calcium-channel blockers	– Uterine relaxation so may inhibit labor – Diltiazem should be avoided – Verapamil may reduce uterine blood flow

Tertiary units should offer a facility to enable women who live some distance away to stay on site, in order to avoid delay in receiving appropriate care when they go into labor, and need to induce labor solely to avoid this risk.

During pregnancy, fetal growth is monitored by the obstetric team and a fetal cardiac echocardiogram is offered at about 22 to 26 weeks to determine whether the baby has a congenital cardiac anomaly.

Atrial fibrillation is rare during pregnancy and is usually associated with another underlying cause, such as mitral stenosis, congenital heart disease, or hyperthyroidism.

Diagnosis and treatment of the underlying condition causing the dysrhythmia is important.

Antithrombotic therapy is recommended for all pregnant women with atrial fibrillation; the type of therapy should be chosen with regard to the stage of pregnancy.

Many women with valvular heart disease can be successfully managed throughout pregnancy, labor, and delivery with conservative medical measures.

Symptomatic or severe valvular lesions should be addressed and rectified before conception and pregnancy whenever possible.

Pregnant women with mild to moderate mitral stenosis can almost always be managed with judicious use of diuretics and beta blockade.

Women with severe mitral stenosis should be considered for percutaneous balloon mitral valvotomy (BMV) before conception, if possible, or during pregnancy.

Mitral regurgitation can usually be managed medically with diuretics and vasodilator therapy.

Pregnant women with mild aortic obstruction and normal left ventricular systolic function can be managed conservatively throughout pregnancy.

Those with moderate to severe obstruction or symptoms should be advised to delay conception until aortic stenosis can be corrected.

Women with severe aortic stenosis who develop symptoms may require percutaneous aortic balloon valvotomy or surgery before labor and delivery.

Isolated aortic regurgitation can usually be managed with diuretics and vasodilator therapy when needed.

Surgery during pregnancy should be contemplated only for control of refractory symptoms; if surgery is required, repair is always preferred.

In patients with mild symptoms and structurally normal hearts, no treatment other than reassurance should be provided.

Given that all commonly used antiarrhythmic drugs cross the placental barrier to some extent, antiarrhythmic drug therapy should be used only if symptoms are intolerable or if the tachycardia causes hemodynamic compromise.

Pregnancy increases the risk for stroke and complicates the selection of acute and preventive treatments.

Recommendations for stroke prevention in pregnant women made by the American Heart Association and American Stroke Association focus on anticoagulation and antiplatelet strategies which are similar to those for management of valvular heart disease during pregnancy.

The 2006 American College of Cardiology and the American Heart Association (ACC/AHA) guidelines on valvular heart disease offer complex recommendations for the management of anticoagulation in pregnant patients with mechanical prosthetic heart valves.

These guidelines reflect high complication rates in pregnant women managed with subcutaneous heparin and support the use of intravenous heparin during the first trimester.

After the 36th week of pregnancy, transition from warfarin to heparin is recommended in anticipation of labor.

Mode of Delivery

Vaginal delivery is the preferred mode of delivery for most women with heart disease, unless there are specific obstetric indications or deterioration in cardiac performance necessitating early delivery.

The rate of caesarean section is much higher for women with heart disease compared with the general population for these reasons.

In most cases, vaginal delivery is best achieved by aiming for spontaneous onset of labor, providing effective pain relief with low-dose regional analgesia and, if necessary, assisting vaginal delivery with instruments such as the ventouse or forceps, in order to limit or avoid maternal effort in 'pushing'.

High-risk patients should be delivered in a center where expertise is available to monitor the hemodynamic changes of labor and delivery, and intervene when necessary.

If vaginal delivery is elected, fetal and maternal ECG monitoring should be performed.

Delivery can be accomplished with the mother in the left lateral position so that the fetus does not compress the inferior vena cava, thereby maintaining venous return.

The second stage should be assisted, if necessary (e.g., forceps or vacuum extraction), to avoid a long labor.

Regional analgesia during labor is usually recommended in order to reduce the further increases in cardiac output and myocardial oxygen demand caused by pain and anxiety; good regional analgesia will also facilitate instrumental delivery.

Induction of labor may be appropriate in order to optimize the timing of delivery in relation to anticoagulation or because of deteriorating maternal cardiac function.

General and regional anaesthesia (spinal, epidural, or combined spinal-epidural) have been used for caesarean section.

A 5 yr review of practice in an Australian hospital found that six of the seven parturients with New York Heart Association (NYHA) grade IV symptoms received regional anaesthesia and 12 out of 17 with NYHA grade III symptoms received regional anaesthesia.

There is no evidence to support any particular technique, but cardiovascular stability is the goal.

Although there is no consensus regarding the administration of antibiotic prophylaxis at the time of delivery for patients with lesions vulnerable to infective endocarditis, many institutions routinely give antibiotics because of the documented bacteremia even during an uncomplicated delivery.

It is recommended that if oxytocin is required post-delivery, it should only be administered by infusion with the omission of a bolus.

It has been argued that the cardiovascular effects of a post-partum haemorrhage in a patient with a fixed cardiac output, and the potential risk of overzealous i.v. fluid replacement in response, are worse than the potential cardiovascular effects of a slow infusion of oxytocin (which include peripheral vasodilation, tachycardia, and fluid retention).

Ergometrine should be avoided in severe cardiac disease as it leads to vasoconstriction and hypertension, and increases the risk of myocardial infarction and pulmonary oedema.

Carboprost is not recommended in cardiac disease as it too has the potential to cause/exacerbate pulmonary oedema.

It should also be noted that the use of a glyceryl trinitrate infusion post-delivery may improve pulmonary oedema; however, it may also increase the risk of post-partum haemorrhage due to uterine relaxation.

Post-partum

In the post-partum period, high-level maternal surveillance is required until the main haemodynamic changes after delivery have resolved.

For particularly unstable cardiac conditions, such surveillance may be required in hospital for up to 2 weeks.

A review of parturients with heart disease found that the worst cardiac compromise did not always occur at the time of delivery.

The occurrence of chest infection or development of peripartum cardiomyopathy (which may occur anytime from 1 month pre-delivery up to 5 months post-delivery) in some cases lead to worse compromise post-delivery.

VALVULAR HEART DISEASE

Valvular heart disease in pregnancy is relatively infrequent, with an incidence of less than 1%.

In the developed world, valvular disease in women of childbearing age is often congenitally acquired.

Rheumatic heart disease, myxomatous degeneration, previous endocarditis, and bicuspid aortic valves are also encountered.

Pregnancy complicated by valvular heart disease tends to have a favorable prognosis if the risks are appropriately managed.

The ACC/AHA classifies maternal and fetal risk during pregnancy based on:

(1) the type of valvular abnormality and

(2) the NYHA functional classification.

High Maternal and Fetal Risk Conditions

- Severe aortic stenosis with or without symptoms
- Aortic regurgitation with NYHA class III or IV symptoms
- Mitral stenosis with NYHA class II, III, or IV symptoms
- Mitral regurgitation with NYHA class III or IV symptoms
- Aortic valve disease, mitral valve disease, or both resulting in pulmonary hypertension with a pulmonary pressure greater than 75% of systemic pressures
- Aortic valve disease, mitral valve disease, or both with left ventricular ejection fraction less than 40%
- Maternal cyanosis
- Any valve disease with NYHA class III or IV symptoms

Low Maternal and Fetal Risk Conditions

– Asymptomatic aortic stenosis with a mean transvalvular gradient of less than 50 mm Hg and normal left ventricular systolic function

– Aortic regurgitation with NYHA class I or II symptoms and normal left ventricular systolic function

– Mitral regurgitation with NYHA class I or II symptoms and normal left ventricular systolic function

– Mitral valve prolapse with no regurgitation or with mild-to-moderate regurgitation and normal left ventricular systolic function

– Mild-to-moderate mitral stenosis (mitral valve area >1.5 cm^2, gradient <5 mm Hg) without severe pulmonary hypertension

– Mild-to-moderate pulmonary valve stenosis

Decreased functional status (NYHA class II or higher) and specific valvular conditions including mitral stenosis and aortic stenosis are associated with increased neonatal complications such as premature birth, intrauterine growth restriction, respiratory distress syndrome, intraventricular hemorrhage, and death.

If medical intervention is necessary during pregnancy, the lowest adequate therapeutic dose of the required medication should be used.

Medications such as hydralazine, methyldopa, digoxin, adenosine, and procainamide can be safely used in pregnancy.

Angiotensin converting enzyme (ACE) inhibitors, angiotensin receptor blockers, amiodarone, and nitroprusside are contraindicated during pregnancy regardless of the indication.

Most other medications carry a potential risk to the fetus and should only be used when the maternal benefit outweighs the fetal risk.

In a woman with valvular disease, a short, pain-free labor and delivery helps to minimize hemodynamic changes.

Hemodynamic monitoring, including continuous monitoring of oxygen saturation, ECG, and arterial pressure should be under surveillance.

Rarely, pulmonary artery wedge pressures, and cardiac output, may be indicated in severe disease.

Fetal monitoring is another means of assessing the adequacy of cardiac treatment because fetal distress is an indicator of impaired cardiac output.

Women with valvular disease should undergo a vaginal delivery with adequate pain control as caesarean delivery results in greater hemodynamic changes and blood loss and should be reserved for obstetric indications.

In certain patients, especially those with mitral or aortic stenosis, delivery should be aided by forceps or vacuum-assisted techniques to avoid the sudden rise in systemic vascular resistance and drop in systemic venous return that occurs with maternal pushing.

Endocarditis prophylaxis remains a controversial issue in vaginal and cesarian deliveries.

The ACC/AHA guidelines recommend against prophylaxis in cesarian deliveries.

In vaginal deliveries, the ACC/AHA does not recommend prophylaxis, but discretion is left to the physician who is caring for high-risk patients.

Early studies reported a low incidence of bacteremia with vaginal delivery.

However, more recent studies found, in some circumstances, the incidence can be as high as 5-19%.

When endocarditis occurs during pregnancy, maternal and fetal mortality rates are 22% and 25%, respectively.

In patients with underlying valvular heart disease, many centers administer prophylaxis antibiotics using the AHA guidelines of ampicillin 2.0 g IM or IV plus gentamicin 1.5 mg/kg (not to exceed 120 mg) given at initiation of labor or within 30 min of a caesarean delivery, followed by ampicillin 1 g IM or IV or amoxicillin 1 g orally6 hours later.

For patients allergic to penicillin, vancomycin 1.0 g IV over 1-2 hours is recommended instead.

MITRAL STENOSIS

The predominant cause of mitral stenosis is rheumatic fever, with rheumatic changes present in 99% of stenotic mitral valves excised at the time of mitral valve replacement.

Other possibilities include congenital mitral stenosis, systemic lupus erythematosus, rheumatoid arthritis, atrial myxoma, malignant carcinoid, and bacterial endocarditis.

About 25% of all patients with rheumatic heart disease have isolated mitral stenosis, and about 40% have combined mitral stenosis and mitral regurgitation.

Rheumatic fever results in characteristic changes of the mitral valve with the diagnostic features being thickening at the leaflet edges, fusion of the commissures, and chordal shortening and fusion with acute rheumatic fever, there is inflammation and edema of the leaflets, with small fibrin-platelet thrombi along the leaflet contact zones.

Subsequent scarring leads to the characteristic valve deformity with obliteration of the normal leaflet architecture by fibrosis, neovascularization and increased collagen and tissue cellularity; superimposed calcification results in further dysfunction.

The pregnancy-induced increase in plasma volume leads to elevated left atrial and pulmonary vein pressures.

This may cause pulmonary edema and lead to symptoms of dyspnea, orthopnea, and paroxysmal nocturnal dyspnea.

The increased heart rate observed during pregnancy, decreases diastolic filling time, which further increases left atrial pressure.

This may provoke atrial arrhythmias, which shortens diastolic filling time even further.

The first bouts of dyspnea in patients with mitral stenosis are usually precipitated by tachycardia resulting from exercise, pregnancy, hyperthyroidism, anemia, infection, or atrial fibrillation, all of which both (1) increase the rate of blood flow across the mitral orifice resulting in further elevation of the left atrial pressure and

(2) decrease the diastolic filling time resulting in a reduction in forward cardiac output.

Pulmonary hypertension in mitral stenosis results from

(1) passive backward transmission of the elevated left atrial pressure;

(2) pulmonary arteriolar constriction, which presumably is triggered by left atrial and pulmonary venous hypertension (reactive pulmonary hypertension); and

(3) organic obliterative changes in the pulmonary vascular bed, which may be considered to be a complication of long standing and severe mitral stenosis.

In time, severe pulmonary hypertension results in right-sided heart failure, with dilation of the right ventricle and its annulus and secondary TR and sometimes pulmonic regurgitation.

The most common presenting symptoms of mitral stenosis are fatigue and decreased exercise tolerance; dyspnea may be accompanied by cough and wheezing.

Patients who have critical obstruction to left atrial emptying and dyspnea with ordinary activity NYHA Class III generally have orthopnea as well and are at risk of experiencing attacks of frank pulmonary edema.

The latter may be precipitated by effort, emotional stress, respiratory infection, fever, sexual intercourse, pregnancy, or atrial fibrillation with a rapid ventricular rate or other tachyarrhythmia.

Hemoptysis is rare in patients with a known diagnosis of mitral stenosis because intervention is performed before severe obstruction becomes chronic.

When hemoptysis does occur it can be sudden and severe, caused by rupture of thin-walled, dilated bronchial veins, usually as a consequence of a sudden rise in left atrial pressure, or it may be milder with only blood-stained sputum associated with attacks of paroxysmal nocturnal dyspnea.

Chest pain is not a typical symptom of mitral stenosis, but a small percentage, perhaps 15%, of patients with mitral stenosis experience chest discomfort that is indistinguishable from angina pectoris.

Rarely, chest pain may be secondary to coronary obstruction caused by coronary embolization.

Echocardiography is the most accurate approach to diagnosis and evaluation of mitral stenosis.

Echocardiography is recommended in all patients with mitral stenosis at initial presentation, for reevaluation of changing symptoms or signs, and at regular intervals (depending on disease severity) for monitoring disease progression.

When transthoracic images are suboptimal, transesophageal echocardiography (TEE) is appropriate.

TEE is also necessary to exclude left atrial thrombus and to evaluate mitral regurgitation severity when percutaneous BMV is considered.

However, mitral valve morphology typically is best evaluated on transthoracic imaging.

Exercise testing is useful in many patients with mitral stenosis to ascertain the level of physical conditioning.

The exercise test can be combined with Doppler echocardiography to assess exercise hemodynamics, usually with the Doppler examination performed at rest after termination of exercise.

Exercise Doppler testing is recommended when there is a discrepancy between resting echocardiographic findings and the severity of clinical symptoms.

In temperate zones, such as the United States and Western Europe, patients who develop acute rheumatic fever have an asymptomatic period of approximately 15-20 years before symptoms of mitral stenosis develop.

It then takes approximately 5-10 years for most patients to progress from mild disability (i.e., early NYHA Class II) to severe disability (i.e., NYHA Class III or IV).

The most likely causes for these differences are the relative prevalence of rheumatic fever, and lack of primary and secondary prevention resulting in recurrent episodes of valve scarring.

There are little data on the rate of hemodynamic progression of rheumatic mitral stenosis in underdeveloped countries where the age at symptom onset is much younger.

Despite the high risk of complications, maternal mortality is generally less than 1% and appears to be confined to patients with severe mitral stenosis and NYHA class IV symptoms.

Fetal complications include preterm delivery and intrauterine growth restriction.

Fetal mortality increases with worsening maternal functional capacity and may be as high as 30% when the mother has NYHA class IV symptoms.

Overall clinical outcomes are greatly improved in patients who undergo surgical or percutaneous relief of valve obstruction on the basis of current guidelines.

The medical management of mitral stenosis is directed toward

(1) prevention of recurrent rheumatic fever,

(2) prevention and treatment of complications of mitral stenosis and

(3) monitoring disease progression to allow intervention at the optimal time point.

Patients with mitral stenosis caused by rheumatic heart disease should receive penicillin prophylaxis for beta-hemolytic streptococcal infections to prevent recurrent rheumatic fever per established guidelines; prophylaxis for infective endocarditis is no longer recommended.

Anemia and infections should be treated promptly and aggressively in patients with valvular heart disease.

However, blood cultures should always be considered before beginning antibiotic therapy in patients with valve disease because the presentation of endocarditis often is mistaken for a non-cardiac infection.

Management of the pregnant woman with mitral stenosis should include reducing the heart rate and left atrial pressure by restricting physical activity and administering a beta-adrenergic receptor blocker.

In patients with atrial fibrillation, digoxin may also be useful as well as safe for control of ventricular rate.

If a calcium channel blocker is needed, verapamil is preferred over diltiazem.

Left atrial pressure can also be reduced by decreasing blood volume through salt restriction and the use of oral diuretics.

Aggressive use of diuretics should be avoided to prevent hypovolemia and reduction of uteroplacental perfusion.

Anticoagulant therapy is indicated for prevention of systemic embolism in mitral stenosis patients with atrial fibrillation (persistent or paroxysmal), any prior embolic events (even if in sinus rhythm) and in those with documented left atrial thrombus.

Anticoagulation also may be considered in patients with severe mitral stenosis and sinus rhythm when there is severe left atrial enlargement (diameter >55 mm) or spontaneous contrast on echocardiography.

Treatment with warfarin is used to maintain the international normalized ratio (INR) between 2 and 3.

Asymptomatic patients with mild to moderate rheumatic mitral valve disease should have a history and physical examination yearly with echocardiography every 3 to 5 years for mild stenosis, every 1 to 2 years for moderate stenosis, and annually for severe stenosis.

Hemoptysis is managed by measures designed to reduce pulmonary venous pressure, including sedation, assumption of the upright position, and aggressive diuresis.

In patients with severe symptoms, percutaneous BMV performed during the second trimester has been associated with normal subsequent deliveries and excellent fetal outcomes.

This procedure is preferable to open mitral valve commissurotomy, which carries a fetal loss rate of 10-30%.

Commissurotomy is reserved for patients with severe mitral stenosis who are refractory to optimal medical therapy and are not suitable candidates for percutaneous BMV.

Mitral valve replacement is recommended for symptomatic patients with severe mitral regurgitation when BMV or surgical mitral valve repair is not possible.

Most often, mitral valve replacement is required in patients with combined mitral stenosis and moderate or severe MR; in those with extensive commissural calcification, severe fibrosis, and subvalvular fusion; and in those who have undergone previous valvotomy.

Prosthetic valves are associated with increased risk because of valve deterioration and chronic anticoagulation.

A mechanical valve is preferred when mitral valve replacement for mitral stenosis is necessary in patients younger than 65 years of age, particularly when atrial fibrillation is present because of the need for chronic anticoagulation.

In patients younger than age 65 who are in sinus rhythm, a mechanical valve is reasonable because of the risk of tissue valve deterioration and likely need for a second operation in the future.

However, some younger patients may choose a bioprosthetic valve for lifestyle considerations, despite the risk of valve deterioration.

A bioprosthetic valve is appropriate in patients who cannot take warfarin and is reasonable in patients older than 65 years of age.

Mitral valve replacement is indicated in two groups of patients with mitral stenosis whose valves are not suitable for valvotomy:

(1) those with a mitral valve area less than 1.5 cm^2 in NYHA Class III or IV; and

(2) those with severe mitral stenosis (mitral valve area <1 cm^2), NYHA Class II, and severe pulmonary hypertension (pulmonary artery systolic pressure >70 mm Hg).

Because the operative mortality risk may be quite high (10-20%) in patients in NYHA Class IV, operation should be carried out before patients reach this stage if possible.

On the other hand, even such high-risk patients should not be denied operation unless they have comorbid conditions that preclude surgery or a satisfactory outcome.

Ultrasound examinations to monitor fetal growth are recommended monthly.

Fetal monitoring with nonstress tests and amniotic fluid levels should be considered in women with poor functional status or during any acute changes in maternal symptoms.

Management in labor usually focuses on avoiding rapid changes in hemodynamic status and avoidance of tachycardia.

Epidural anesthesia is useful in avoiding the catecholamine-induced tachycardia.

Epidural anesthesia is usually preferred over spinal anesthesia because it has a slower onset of blockade and therefore more controlled hemodynamic changes.

Vaginal delivery is usually well tolerated; caesarean delivery should be performed for obstetrical indications only, as the hemodynamic changes from caesarean delivery may be more detrimental postpartum than those that occur during vaginal delivery.

MITRAL REGURGITATION

The mitral valve apparatus involves the mitral leaflets, chordae tendineae, papillary muscles, and mitral annulus; abnormalities of any of these structures may cause mitral regurgitation.

Mitral regurgitation in pregnancy is usually due to mitral valve prolapse or rheumatic heart disease.

Other causes include infective endocarditis, annular calcification, cardiomyopathy, and ischemic heart disease.

Less common causes of mitral regurgitation include collagen vascular diseases, trauma, the hypereosinophilic syndrome, carcinoid, and exposure to certain drugs.

Idiopathic (degenerative) calcification of the mitral annulus is one of the most common cardiac abnormalities found at autopsy.

Annular calcification may also be accelerated by an intrinsic defect in the fibrous skeleton of the heart, as in Marfan and Hurler syndromes.

In these two latter syndromes, the mitral annulus is not only calcified but also dilated, further contributing to mitral regurgitation.

In most patients with severe primary mitral regurgitation, compensation is maintained for years, but in some patients the prolonged hemodynamic overload ultimately leads to myocardial decompensation.

End-systolic volume, preload, and afterload all rise, whereas ejection fraction and stroke volume decline.

Preoperative myocardial contractility is an important determinant of the risk of operative death, of cardiac failure perioperatively, and of the level of left ventricle function postoperatively.

Therefore it is not surprising that the end-systolic pressure/volume (or stress/dimension) relation has emerged as a useful index for evaluating left ventricle function in patients with mitral regurgitation.

In patients with rheumatic mitral regurgitation, the time interval between the initial attack of rheumatic fever and the development of symptoms tends to be longer than in those with mitral stenosis and often exceeds two decades.

Hemoptysis and systemic embolization are less common in patients with isolated mitral regurgitation than in those with mitral stenosis.

The development of atrial fibrillation affects the course adversely but perhaps not as dramatically as in mitral stenosis.

On the other hand, chronic weakness and fatigue secondary to a low cardiac output are more prominent features in mitral regurgitation.

Exercise echocardiography is helpful in determining severity of mitral regurgitation and hemodynamic abnormalities (such as pulmonary hypertension) during exercise.

This is a useful, objective means to evaluate symptoms in patients who appear to have only mild mitral regurgitation at rest and to determine functional status in patients who otherwise appear asymptomatic.

Doppler echocardiography in mitral regurgitation characteristically reveals a high-velocity jet in the left atrium during systole.

The severity of the regurgitation is reflected in the width of the jet across the valve and the size of the left atrium.

Natural history of mitral regurgitation is highly variable and depends on a combination of the volume of regurgitation, state of the myocardium, and the cause of the underlying disorder.

Asymptomatic patients with mild mitral regurgitation usually remain in a stable state for many years.

Severe regurgitation develops in only a small percentage of these patients, most commonly because of intervening infective endocarditis or rupture of the chordae tendineae.

Atrial fibrillation is a common arrhythmia is patients with chronic mitral regurgitation, associated with age and left atrial dilation, and its onset is a marker for disease progression.

Patients with atrial fibrillation have an adverse outcome compared to patients who remain in sinus rhythm, and development of atrial fibrillation is considered an indication for operative intervention.

It is usually well tolerated during pregnancy due to the decrease in systemic vascular resistance; asymptomatic patients do not require specific therapy during pregnancy.

In the presence of symptomatic left ventricular dysfunction with hemodynamic abnormalities, diuretics, digoxin, hydralazine, and nitrates can be administered.

The role of pharmacological therapy for mitral regurgitation remains another subject of uncertainty and some debate.

Although there is no doubt that afterload reduction therapy is indicated, and indeed may be lifesaving, in patients with acute MR, the indications for such therapy in patients with chronic mitral regurgitation are much less clear.

Surgery for mitral valve repair or replacement during pregnancy has been associated with a high incidence of fetal loss.

Surgical treatment should be considered for patients with functional disability and/or for patients with no symptoms or only mild symptoms but with progressively deteriorating left ventricle function or progressively increasing left ventricle dimensions as documented by noninvasive studies.

Without surgical treatment, the prognosis for patients with mitral regurgitation and heart failure is poor, and hence mitral valve repair or replacement is indicated in symptomatic patients.

When operative treatment is being considered, the chronic and often slowly but progressive nature of mitral regurgitation must be weighed against the immediate risks and long-term uncertainties attendant upon surgery, especially if mitral valve replacement is required.

Surgical mortality depends on the patient's clinical and hemodynamic status (particularly the function of the left ventricle); on the patient's age; on the presence of comorbid conditions such as renal, hepatic, or pulmonary disease; and on the skill and experience of the surgical team.

The decision to replace or to repair the valve is of critical importance, and mitral valve repair is strongly recommended whenever possible.

Replacement involves the operative risk, as well as the risks of thrombo-embolism and anticoagulation in patients receiving mechanical prostheses, of late structural valve deterioration in patients receiving bioprostheses, and of late mortality.

Surgical mortality does not depend significantly on which of the currently used tissue or mechanical valve prostheses is selected.

Preoperative atrial fibrillation is an independent predictor of reduced long-term survival after mitral valve surgery for chronic mitral regurgitation.

The persistence of atrial fibrillation postoperatively requires long-term anticoagulation, thereby partially nullifying the advantages of mitral valve repair.

Although mitral valve replacement has been used successfully in treating mitral regurgitation for almost four decades, there has been some dissatisfaction with the results of this operation.

First, left ventricle function often deteriorates following mitral valve replacement, leading to early and late mortality and late disability.

A second disadvantage of mitral valve replacement is the prosthesis itself, including the risks of thromboembolism or hemorrhage associated with mechanical prostheses, late structural deterioration of bioprostheses, and infective endocarditis with all prostheses.

For these reasons, increasing efforts are being made to repair the mitral valve whenever possible in patients with isolated or predominant mitral regurgitation.

A large proportion of operative survivors have improved clinical status, quality of life, and exercise tolerance following mitral valve repair or replacement.

However, patients with mitral regurgitation who have marked left ventricle dysfunction preoperatively sometimes remain symptomatic with depressed left ventricle function; progressive left ventricle dysfunction and death from heart failure may occur.

Thus every effort should be made to operate on patients before they develop serious symptoms, and even asymptomatic patients with severe mitral regurgitation may be considered for surgery in an experienced center if there is a high likelihood (>90%) that the valve can be repaired successfully without residual mitral regurgitation.

AORTIC STENOSIS

Obstruction to left ventricular outflow is localized most commonly at the aortic valve.

However, obstruction may also occur above the valve (supravalvular stenosis) or below the valve, or it may be caused by hypertrophic cardiomyopathy.

Valvular aortic stenosis has three principal causes: a congenital bicuspid valve with superimposed calcification, calcification of a normal trileaflet valve (e.g. "degenerative aortic stenosis") and rheumatic disease.

Rheumatic aortic stenosis results from adhesions and fusions of the commissures and cusps and vascularization of the leaflets of the valve ring, leading to retraction and stiffening of the free borders of the cusps.

Calcific nodules develop on both surfaces, and the orifice is reduced to a small round or triangular opening.

An aortic valve orifice of 1.0 to 1.5 cm^2 is considered moderate stenosis, and an orifice of 1.5 to 2.0 cm^2 is referred to as mild stenosis.

However, the degree of stenosis associated with symptom onset varies between patients and there is no single number that defines severe or critical aortic stenosis in an individual patient.

Chronic pressure overload typically results in concentric left ventricle hypertrophy with increased wall thickness and a normal chamber size.

Systemic vascular resistance also contributes to total left ventricle afterload in adults with aortic stenosis.

Concurrent hypertension increases total ventricular load and may affect the evaluation of aortic stenosis severity.

The cardinal manifestations of acquired aortic stenosis are exertional dyspnea, angina pectoris, syncope, and ultimately heart failure.

Many patients now are diagnosed before symptom onset on the basis of the finding of a systolic murmur on physical examination with confirmation of the diagnosis by echocardiography.

Angina occurs in approximately two thirds of patients with severe aortic stenosis (associated significant coronary artery obstruction).

Syncope is most commonly due to reduced cerebral perfusion with severe aortic stenosis.

Other late findings in isolated aortic stenosis include atrial fibrillation, pulmonary hypertension, and systemic venous hypertension.

Echocardiographic imaging allows accurate definition of valve anatomy including the cause of aortic stenosis and the severity of valve calcification and sometimes allows direct imaging of the orifice area.

Echocardiographic imaging also is invaluable for evaluation of left ventricle hypertrophy and systolic function, with calculation of ejection fraction, as well as for measurement of aortic root dimensions and detection of associated mitral valve disease.

Doppler echocardiography allows measurement of the transaortic jet velocity, which is the most useful measure for following disease severity and predicting clinical outcome.

Effective orifice area is calculated using the continuity equation, and mean transaortic pressure gradient can be calculated using the modified Bernoulli equation.

Once even mild symptoms are present, survival is poor unless outflow obstruction is relieved.

Survival curves derived from older retrospective studies show that the interval from the onset of symptoms to the time of death is approximately 2 years in patients with heart failure, 3 years in those with syncope, and 5 years in those with angina.

More recent series confirm this poor prognosis with an average survival of only 1 to 3 years after symptom onset.

The most important principle in management of aortic stenosis is patient education regarding the disease course and typical symptoms.

Patients should be advised to report promptly the development of any symptoms possibly related to aortic stenosis.

Patients with severe aortic stenosis should be cautioned to avoid vigorous athletic and physical activity; however, such restrictions do not apply to patients with mild obstruction.

Evolving recommendations for infective endocarditis prophylaxis should be explained.

Echocardiography is recommended for initial diagnosis and assessment of aortic stenosis severity, for assessment of left ventricle hypertrophy and systolic function, for reevaluation in patients with changing signs or symptoms, and for reevaluation annually for severe aortic stenosis, every 1-2 years for moderate aortic stenosis, and every 3 to 5 years for mild aortic stenosis.

Most patients with mild aortic stenosis have a favorable outcome; moderate-to-severe stenosis has an increased risk of cardiac and obstetrical complications.

Cardiac complications in patients with aortic stenosis include heart failure (7%), arrhythmias (2.5%), and ischemic events (2.5%).

The increased cardiac output related to pregnancy can lead to heart failure, and the increased heart rate in the third trimester can lead to ischemic events.

The potential obstetrical complications include preeclampsia or other hypertensive related disorders, premature birth, and small-for-gestational-age births.

These patients should be followed closely in the third trimester, including ultrasound to monitor fetal growth.

Patients with congenital aortic valve stenosis have increased risk of congenital heart disease in the fetus of 4%; these patients may benefit from fetal echocardiography at 20-22 weeks.

Symptomatic patients with severe aortic stenosis are usually operative candidates because medical therapy has little to offer.

However, medical therapy may be necessary in patients who are considered to be inoperable.

ACE inhibitors should be used with caution but are beneficial in treating patients with symptomatic left ventricle systolic dysfunction who are not candidates for surgery.

They should be initiated at low doses and increased slowly to target doses, avoiding hypotension.

Beta-adrenergic blockers can depress myocardial function and induce left ventricle failure and should be avoided in patients with aortic stenosis.

Adults with asymptomatic severe aortic stenosis can undergo pregnancy with careful hemodynamic monitoring and optimization of loading conditions.

However, when stenosis is very severe, elective aortic valve replacement prior to a planned pregnancy may be considered.

In the adolescent or young adult with severe congenital aortic stenosis, balloon aortic valvotomy is recommended in all symptomatic patients and in asymptomatic patients with a transvalvular gradient greater than 60 mm Hg or ECG ST changes at rest or with exercise.

Aortic valve replacement is recommended in adults with symptomatic severe aortic stenosis, even if symptoms are mild.

Aortic valve replacement also is recommended for severe aortic stenosis with an ejection fraction less than 50% and in patients with severe asymptomatic aortic stenosis who are undergoing coronary bypass grafting or other heart surgery.

Surgical risk is higher in patients with impaired left ventricle function (EF <35%).

However, their prognosis is extremely poor without operation, overall survival is improved with aortic valve replacement, and many patients in this group have significant clinical and functional recovery following aortic valve replacement; hence it should generally be offered to these patients.

Anesthesia management at delivery is controversial because patients may not tolerate the decrease in preload and afterload that occurs with regional anesthesia.

Labor is not contraindicated; an assisted second stage is appropriate to minimize significant changes in the cardiac output that can occur during prolonged labor.

Ideally, women with symptomatic aortic stenosis should have surgical intervention prior to pregnancy.

Some experts offer pregnancy termination in the face of symptomatic severe aortic stenosis; the patient should be counseled about the maternal risks of pregnancy.

AORTIC REGURGITATION

Aortic regurgitation may be caused by primary disease of the aortic valve leaflets and/or the wall of the aortic root.

Primary valvular causes of aortic regurgitation include calcific aortic stenosis in the elderly, in which some degree (usually mild) of aortic regurgitation is present in 75% of patients; infective endocarditis (in which the infection may destroy or cause perforation of a leaflet, or the vegetations may interfere with proper coaptation of the cusps; and trauma that results in a tear of the ascending aorta.

Rheumatic fever remains a common cause of primary disease of the aortic valve that leads to regurgitation.

The cusps become infiltrated with fibrous tissues and retract, a process that prevents cusp apposition during diastole and usually leads to regurgitation into the left ventricle through a defect in the valve.

AR, regardless of its cause, produces dilation and hypertrophy of the left ventricle, dilation of the mitral valve ring, and sometimes hypertrophy and dilation of the left atrium.

Endocardial pockets frequently develop in the left ventricle cavity at sites of impact of the regurgitant jet.

In aortic regurgitation there is an increase in both preload and afterload; left ventricle systolic function is maintained through the combination of chamber dilation and hypertrophy.

In patients with chronic, severe aortic regurgitation, the left ventricle gradually enlarges while the patient remains asymptomatic.

Symptoms of reduced cardiac reserve or myocardial ischemia develop, most often in the fourth or fifth decade and usually only after considerable cardiomegaly and myocardial dysfunction have occurred.

The principal complaints of exertional dyspnea, orthopnea, and paroxysmal nocturnal dyspnea usually develop gradually.

Angina pectoris is prominent late in the course; nocturnal angina may be troublesome.

Patients with severe aortic regurgitation often complain of an uncomfortable awareness of the heartbeat, especially on lying down, and thoracic pain due to pounding of the heart against the chest wall.

Tachycardia, occurring with emotional stress or exertion, may cause troubling palpitations and head pounding; premature ventricular contractions are particularly distressing.

Echocardiography is helpful in identifying the cause of aortic regurgitation and may demonstrate a bicuspid valve, thickening of the valve cusps, other congenital abnormalities, prolapse of the valve, a flail leaflet, or vegetation.

Transthoracic echocardiography is useful for the measurement of left ventricle end-diastolic and end-systolic dimensions and volumes, ejection fraction, and mass.

Doppler echocardiography and color flow Doppler imaging are the most sensitive and accurate noninvasive techniques in the diagnosis and evaluation of aortic regurgitation.

They readily detect mild degrees of aortic regurgitation that may be inaudible on physical examination.

Both the aortic regurgitant orifice size and the aortic regurgitant flow can be estimated quantitatively and are strongly recommended.

These quantitative data provide the basis for the definitions of mild, moderate, and severe.

Moderate or even severe chronic aortic regurgitation may be associated with a generally favorable prognosis for many years.

Among asymptomatic patients with severe aortic regurgitation and normal left ventricle ejection fractions, more than 45% remain asymptomatic with normal left ventricle function at 10 years.

Recommendations for antibiotic prophylaxis for infective endocarditis have changed recently, and the majority of patients with aortic regurgitation are not candidates for prophylaxis.

Patients with mild or moderate aortic regurgitation who are asymptomatic with normal or only minimally increased cardiac size require no therapy but should be followed clinically and by echocardiography every 12 or 24 months.

Asymptomatic patients with chronic, severe aortic regurgitation and normal left ventricle function should be examined at intervals of approximately 6 months.

However, patients with aortic regurgitation who have limitations of cardiac reserve and/or evidence of declining left ventricle function should not engage in vigorous sports or heavy exertion.

Systemic arterial diastolic hypertension, if present, should be treated.

Aortic valve replacement is the treatment of choice in symptomatic patients; chronic medical therapy may be necessary in some patients who refuse surgery or are considered to be inoperable because of comorbid conditions.

These patients should receive an aggressive heart failure regimen with ACE inhibitors (and perhaps other vasodilators), digoxin, diuretics, and salt restriction, but beta blockers should be avoided.

Even though nitroglycerin and other nitrates are not as helpful in relieving anginal pain in patients with aortic regurgitation as they are in coronary artery disease or aortic stenosis, they are worth a try.

In the absence of obvious contraindications or serious comorbidity, surgical treatment is advisable for symptomatic patients with severe aortic regurgitation and for asymptomatic patients with an ejection fraction less than 50% and severe left ventricle dilation (end-diastolic diameter >75 mm or end-systolic diameter ≥55 mm).

As is true for patients with aortic stenosis, the operative risk of aortic valve replacement for patients with aortic regurgitation depends on the general condition of the patient, the state of left ventricle function, and the skill and experience of the surgical team.

The mortality rate ranges from 3-8% in most medical centers; late mortality of approximately 5-10% per year is observed in survivors who had marked cardiac enlargement and/or prolonged left ventricle dysfunction preoperatively.

By extending the indications for operation to symptomatic patients with normal left ventricle function, as well as to asymptomatic patients with left ventricle dysfunction, both early and late results are improving.

PROSTHETIC HEART VALVES

Risks of prosthetic heart valves in pregnant patient include thromboembolism, structural valve failure, bleeding secondary to anticoagulation, and infection.

Women with mechanical prosthetic heart valves require lifelong anticoagulation to prevent valve thrombosis.

Women with bioprosthetic valves do not require anticoagulation; however, some theoretical concern exists that the increased blood volume associated with pregnancy may hasten valve deterioration.

Overall, the durability of bioprosthetic valves is about 10 years and has not be shown to be less in women who have had pregnancies.

Valve thrombosis is a life-threatening condition, and, therefore, women with mechanical prosthetic valves require anticoagulation.

Warfarin crosses the placenta, and its use is associated with embryopathy, fetal loss, and fetal cerebral hemorrhage.

The ACC/AHA guidelines suggest using unfractionated heparin or low molecular weight heparin (LMWH) from 6-12 weeks of gestation and then conversion back to warfarin until 36 weeks of gestation, at which time women are converted back to heparin or LMWH.

The 2008 American College of Chest Physicians guidelines support maintaining LMWH as a treatment option in these women.

Treatment options including risks and benefits to both mother and fetus should be discussed with the patient, and patient preference is an important part of the decision.

However, much debate has occurred regarding the use of LMWH in pregnancy due to a suspected increased risk of valve thrombosis.

Recent studies have shown that rates of thromboembolic events are low if LMWH dosing is adjusted according to anti-factor Xa levels.

If LMWH is to be used in pregnancy, women are recommended to receive 1mg/kg twice daily, and anti-factor Xa levels are followed with a goal of 1.0-1.2 U/ml 4-6 hours after injection.

Preconceptually, patients should be counseled to continue warfarin until pregnancy is confirmed.

Early diagnosis of pregnancy is important to decrease the fetal risks of warfarin.

Patients should be converted to unfractionated heparin or LMWH in the first trimester as soon as pregnancy is determined.

Timing of delivery should be anticipated so that anticoagulation can be managed to decrease the risk of bleeding.

If urgent delivery is necessary while receiving warfarin, reversal of anticoagulation is appropriate to avoid massive hemorrhage; however, the benefit must be weighed against risk of thrombosis.

CONGENITAL HEART DISEASE

With advances in management of congenital heart disease, almost 85% of patients with congenital heart disease now survive to adulthood and childbearing age.

Traditionally, these patients were advised against pregnancy; however, as our understanding of the unique issues facing this population has improved, many of those limitations have been removed.

Although some patients with congenital heart disease may not tolerate the hemodynamic changes of pregnancy, many women have sufficient cardiac reserve to safely carry a pregnancy to term.

Death is a rare occurrence during pregnancy in women with congenital heart disease; however, maternal and fetal complications are substantial.

The risk of the infant having a congenital abnormality ranges from an average of 3% to about 50% in autosomal dominant single gene defects such as Marfan syndrome.

Simple lesions with minimal hemodynamic changes, such as small atrial septal defects, carry a low risk of maternal deterioration or fetal complications.

On the other hand, Eisenmenger syndrome carries a significant risk of deterioration to the mother including death.

Cyanotic congenital heart diseases carry the highest risk to the fetus, from intrauterine growth restriction to spontaneous abortion.

Management should start early with preconception risk stratification using appropriate clinical and laboratory investigations.

Emphasis should be placed on the risk factors that are highlighted below:

High Maternal Risk Factors

– Poor functional class before pregnancy (NYHA II or more) or cyanosis

– Impaired systemic ventricular function (ejection fraction <40%)

– Mitral valve stenosis (area <2 cm^2), aortic valve stenosis (area <1.5 cm^2), left ventricular outflow tract peak pressure gradient greater than 30 mm Hg before pregnancy

– Preconception history of adverse cardiac events such as symptomatic arrhythmia, stroke, transient ischemic attack, and pulmonary edema

– Marfan syndrome

– Eisenmenger syndrome

– Pulmonary hypertension

Moderate Maternal Risk Factors

– Repaired tetralogy of Fallot without significant pulmonic stenosis or regurgitation

– Complex congenital heart disease with the anatomic right ventricle serving as systemic ventricle

– Mild mitral or aortic valve stenosis

– Cyanotic lesions without pulmonary hypertension

– Fontan type circulation

– Uncorrected coarctation of the aorta

Low Maternal Risk Factors

– Small ventricular septal defects

– Atrial septal defects

– Bicuspid aortic valve without stenosis, regurgitation, or aortic dilation

– Repaired coarctation of the aorta

The patient should be informed about multiple issues, including the expected rate of complications and risk of congenital anomalies in her offspring.

Fetal ultrasonographic screening should be offered, with level II ultrasound at 17-18 weeks and fetal echocardiography at 18-22 weeks.

Patients at low risk should receive routine obstetric care and endocarditis prophylaxis as indicated.

Patients at moderate risk usually tolerate pregnancy well; however, they do pose certain management difficulties.

Significant anomalies should be assessed for possible repair prior to pregnancy, and medical management should be modified to avoid certain harmful effects to the fetus.

High-risk patients should be counseled against pregnancy, and, in the event of pregnancy, offering early termination should be considered.

Both moderate-risk and high-risk patients should be followed at tertiary centers with maternal fetal specialists who have extensive experience in dealing with pregnancy in congenital heart disease.

Women with moderate-risk or high-risk lesions, especially cyanotic lesions, have an increased risk of fetal growth restriction and should be followed with monthly ultrasound examinations for fetal growth.

If growth restriction occurs, then these pregnancies need to be followed with twice-weekly NSTs and weekly evaluation of amniotic fluid volumes.

In cases of maternal decompensation, fetal monitoring should also be performed to ensure fetal well being.

Close collaboration between both cardiac and obstetric teams is needed for optimal care.

Decisions about timing and mode of delivery must be made well in advance of labor.

Vaginal delivery is preferred because it causes smaller shifts in blood volume, less hemorrhage, fewer clots, and fewer infections; caesarean delivery is indicated only for obstetric reasons.

Oxygen should be administered to all hypoxemic patients with arterial saturation monitoring for patients with cyanotic conditions, pulmonary hypertension, and cardiac dysfunction.

Hemodynamic monitoring with arterial lines or Swan-Ganz catheters can be performed if necessary.

Epidural anesthesia with adequate volume preloading is the preferred method for labor anesthesia, except in defects when a decrease in systemic vascular resistance is hazardous.

Endocarditis prophylaxis is controversial; the AHA guidelines suggest that prophylaxis is unnecessary except in cases of prosthetic heart valves or surgically constructed systemic to pulmonary shunts.

Due to the devastating effects of endocarditis, some clinicians recommend prophylaxis in vaginal deliveries except in patients with isolated secundum type of atrial septal defect or those who are more than 6 months from surgical repair of septal defects or surgical ligation of patent ductus arteriosus.

ATRIAL SEPTAL DEFECTS

Atrial septal defect (ASD) is one of the more commonly recognized congenital cardiac anomalies presenting in adulthood.

Atrial septal defect is characterized by a defect in the interatrial septum allowing pulmonary venous return from the left atrium to pass directly to the right atrium.

Depending on the size of the defect, size of the shunt, and associated anomalies, this can result in a spectrum of disease from no significant cardiac sequelae to right-sided volume overload, pulmonary arterial hypertension, and even atrial arrhythmias.

With the routine use of echocardiography, the incidence of atrial septal defect is increased compared to earlier incidence studies using catheterization, surgery, or autopsy for diagnosis.

The subtle physical examination findings and often minimal symptoms contribute to a delay in diagnosis until adulthood; however, earlier intervention is recommended.

Atrial septal defects are usually well tolerated during pregnancy; cardiac deterioration occurred more frequently in patients who did not undergo surgical correction of their defect prior to pregnancy.

Generally, decisions concerning pregnancy in this group should be made on an individual basis considering functional status, pulmonary hypertension, and the presence of additional cardiac lesions.

VENTRICULAR SEPTAL DEFECTS

A ventricular septal defect (VSD) is a hole or a defect in the septum that divides the 2 lower chambers of the heart, resulting in communication between the ventricular cavities.

A VSD may occur as a primary anomaly, with or without additional major associated cardiac defects.

It may also occur as a single component of a wide variety of intracardiac anomalies, including tetralogy of Fallot, complete atrioventricular canal defects, transposition of great arteries, and corrected transpositions.

Isolated small VSD are usually well tolerated; however, larger defects are associated with an increased risk of congestive heart failure, arrhythmias, and pulmonary hypertension.

The incidence of occurrence of of VSD in the offspring ranges from 4-11%.

Closure of the VSD prior to the onset of pulmonary hypertension or ventricular dysfunction reduces the incidence of complications to that of the general population.

In patients with pulmonary hypertension, shunt reversal and cyanosis can occur secondary to reduced blood pressure during pregnancy and delivery.

These patients may require vasopressors and close monitoring throughout their pregnancy.

PATENT DUCTUS ARTERIOSUS

Patent ductus arteriosus (PDA), in which there is a persistent communication between the descending thoracic aorta and the pulmonary artery that results from failure of normal physiologic closure of the fetal ductus, is one of the more common congenital heart defects.

Although frequently diagnosed in infants, the discovery of this condition may be delayed until childhood or even adulthood.

In isolated PDA, signs and symptoms are consistent with left-to-right shunting.

Patent ductus arteriosus may also exist with other cardiac anomalies, which must be considered at the time of diagnosis.

In many cases, the diagnosis and treatment of a PDA is critical for survival in neonates with severe obstructive lesions to either the right or left side of the heart.

Outcome of PDA in pregnancy with left-to-right shunting is usually favorable.

However, clinical deterioration and congestive heart failure have been reported.

The incidence of occurrence of PDA in the offspring is less than 1%.

In patients with pulmonary hypertension, reversal of the shunt with cyanosis can occur due to decreased blood pressure and may be prevented by the use of vasopressors.

COARCTATION OF THE AORTA

Coarctation of the aorta is a relatively common defect that accounts for 5-8% of all congenital heart defects.

Coarctation of the aorta may occur as an isolated defect or in association with various other lesions, most commonly bicuspid aortic valve and ventricular septal defect.

The diagnosis of coarctation of the aorta may be missed unless an index of suspicion is maintained, and diagnosis is often delayed until the patient develops congestive heart failure (CHF), which is common in infants, or hypertension, which is common in older children.

Coarctation of the aorta is usually well tolerated in pregnancy; severe hypertension, heart failure, and aortic dissection have been reported.

Complications are less likely in cases of repaired coarctation; however, hypertension is still common, especially with the presence of increased coarctation gradient.

Aortic dissection has been reported in pregnant patients with repaired coarctation.

The incidence of congenital heart disease in the offspring is reported to be 3-4%.

Beta-blockers are the treatment of choice for hypertension in this group of patients due to the added effect of protection against aortic dissection.

TETRALOGY OF FALLOT

Tetralogy of Fallot, which is one of the most common congenital heart disorders, comprises right ventricular outflow tract obstruction (infundibular stenosis), ventricular septal defect, aorta dextroposition, and right ventricular hypertrophy.

The mortality rate in untreated patients reaches 50% by age 6 years, but in the present era of cardiac surgery, children with simple forms of tetralogy of Fallot enjoy good long-term survival with an excellent quality of life.

In uncorrected tetralogy of Fallot, the fall in systemic vascular resistance associated with pregnancy may lead exacerbate the right-to-left shunt.

Poor prognostic factors include maternal hematocrit above 60%, arterial oxygen saturation below 80%, elevated right ventricular systolic pressure and syncopal episodes.

Cyanosis is associated with an increased rate of spontaneous abortion, preterm delivery, and intrauterine growth restriction.

Full surgical correction reduces the risk of complications to that of the general population and, therefore, is recommended prior to conception.

Palliative procedures with residual pulmonic regurgitation, right ventricular dilation and dysfunction, and right ventricular outflow obstruction are risk factors for arrhythmia and heart failure during pregnancy.

Close hemodynamic and arterial saturation monitoring during delivery are recommended for cyanotic or symptomatic patients.

The incidence of congenital heart disease is reported to be 3-17% of offspring.

Complications during pregnancy include maternal arrhythmia, heart failure, and myocardial infarction; a higher rate of preterm delivery and growth restriction also exists.

Women who have undergone repair for transposition of the great vessels are generally advised that pregnancy is safe, but a multidisciplinary approach is needed.

Women who have undergone a Fontan procedure have in the past been advised to avoid pregnancy.

With increasing reports of successful pregnancies, this recommendation is being challenged by some.

Women who were born with complex congenital cardiac lesions such as transposition of the great vessels, tricuspid atresia, and single ventricle are now reaching reproductive age due to the success of Mustard, Senning, or Fontan procedures; multiple studies have reported successful pregnancies in these patients.

EISENMENGER SYNDROME

Eisenmenger syndrome refers to any untreated congenital cardiac defect with intracardiac communication that leads to pulmonary hypertension, reversal of flow, and cyanosis.

The previous left-to-right shunt is converted into a right-to-left shunt secondary to elevated pulmonary artery pressures and associated pulmonary vascular disease.

Lesions in Eisenmenger syndrome, such as large septal defects, are characterized by high pulmonary pressure and/or a high pulmonary flow state.

Eisenmenger syndrome is usually associated with increased maternal morbidity and mortality reaching 40%, usually occurring between the first days and a few weeks after deliver.

Fetal loss, preterm delivery, intrauterine growth restriction, and perinatal death are also more frequent.

Patients in this group should be advised against pregnancy and, in the event of accidental pregnancy, early abortion can be offered.

In patients who chose to continue with their pregnancy, close management by experts is essential.

Early hospitalization to restrict activity and ensure close monitoring may be necessary.

Spontaneous vaginal delivery with continuous hemodynamic monitoring is preferred.

Due to the possibility of prolonged induction and the need for an emergency caesarean delivery, a planned caesarean delivery may be considered.

CARDIOMYOPATHY

HYPERTROPHIC CARDIOMYOPATHY

Hypertrophic cardiomyopathy (HCM) has been considered a relatively rare disease in pregnant women.

However, the diagnosis is increasing in frequency due to increased awareness and improved screening.

HCM may be identified by a systolic ejection heart murmur that increases with Valsalva maneuver, by increased QRS voltage on the ECG, and/or by abnormal wall thickness and Doppler blood flow by echocardiography.

Clinical presentation of this disease is widely variable and pregnancy may increase the morbidity and mortality associated with this condition.

Syncope may occur from left ventricular outflow tract obstruction, arrhythmias, or myocardial ischemia or infarction.

Baseline functional status of the patient is an important determinant of the clinical outcome of these women during pregnancy.

Clinical deterioration during pregnancy is uncommon, occurring in less than 5% of previously asymptomatic patients.

The presence of outflow obstruction at baseline increases the risk of clinical deterioration.

The incidence of arrhythmias and syncope were not found to be increased during pregnancy.

Management of HCM in pregnancy should focus on preventing blood loss and avoiding the use of drugs that cause vasodilatation.

Beta-blockers, diuretics, and calcium channel blockers should be used in patients with symptoms of elevated left ventricular filling pressure.

Patients with history of syncope or life-threatening arrhythmias should be assessed for implantation of an automatic defibrillator.

Vaginal delivery is preferred; shortening of the second stage of labor by the use of forceps or vacuum assistance should be considered in patients with left ventricular outflow obstruction.

Oxytocin is the preferred agent for induction as compared to prostaglandins due to the vasodilatory effect of the latter.

PERIPARTUM CARDIOMYOPATHY

Peripartum cardiomyopathy is a rare disorder with incidence ranging between 1 in 1,485 live births to 1 in 15,000 live births.

Peripartum cardiomyopathy is defined as the development of heart failure in the last month of pregnancy or in the first 5 months after delivery without any identifiable etiology and with objective assessment of left ventricular dysfunction.

If any pregnant or post-partum woman has unexpected and persistent dyspnoea or is noted to be unusually tachypnoeic or tachycardic, and pulmonary embolus has been excluded, she may have peripartum cardiomyopathy and should be investigated further by a cardiologist and usually by echocardiography.

Risk factors associated with peripartum cardiomyopathy are maternal age older than 30 years, gestational hypertension, and twin pregnancies.

The association with gestational hypertension suggests a causal relationship; however, a study performed in women with preeclampsia revealed no change in left ventricular systolic function.

An autoimmune mechanism has been suggested on the basis of high titers of autoantibodies against human cardiac tissue proteins in the sera of patients with peripartum cardiomyopathy that are absent in patients with idiopathic cardiomyopathy.

More evidence supports myocarditis as the possible cause than other suggested etiologies.

Therapy should follow general heart failure guidelines for pregnancy, keeping fetal safety in mind during pregnancy and breastfeeding.

Angiotensin converting enzyme (ACE) inhibitors and angiotensin receptor blockers are contraindicated during pregnancy because of the risk of fetal renal agenesis; usual treatments rely on furosemide and nitrates or hydralazine.

No reliable predictors exist for which of these patients may progress rapidly to need for heart transplant and which may substantively recover.

During pregnancy, IV nitrates and/or hydralazine are often used; after delivery, ACE inhibitors may be initiated.

Amlodipine has also been found to be beneficial in nonischemic cardiomyopathy and may have anti-inflammatory effects, adding extra benefit in peripartum cardiomyopathy.

Beta-receptor antagonists in dilated cardiomyopathy are safe and are not contraindicated in pregnancy, yet, due to the lack of studies in peripartum cardiomyopathy, initiation of this group of medications in the postpartum period seems to be a reasonable approach in patients who continue to have symptoms.

Peripartum cardiomyopathy is associated with increased maternal and fetal risk.

With improved therapy and awareness, the trend is toward better prognosis; a recent study reported an in-hospital mortality of 1.36%, with a total mortality of 2.1%, which is a considerable improvement over previously reported mortality rates of 7-18%.

The course of peripartum cardiomyopathy seems to differ from that of traditional cardiomyopathy with normalization of left ventricular dysfunction occurring in about 50% of patients within 6 months after delivery.

Normalization of cardiac function was more likely in patients with left ventricular ejection fraction more than 30% at the time of diagnosis.

An important clinical issue is the patient's ability to have future pregnancies.

Future pregnancies should be discouraged in patients who do not recover their left ventricular function.

The risk of heart failure and death in women with persistently decreased left ventricular function may be as high as 20% with subsequent pregnancy.

Women with normalization of their left ventricular function (ejection fraction >50%) appear to have better outcomes than those with persistently depressed systolic function.

Nevertheless, they do have a risk of heart failure symptoms and a significant drop in left ventricular ejection fraction with subsequent pregnancies.

In patients with normalization of left ventricular function following delivery, subsequent pregnancies should be managed at high-risk centers.

Coronary artery disease should be considered, particularly if a family history of early atherosclerotic disease exists, or other risk factors such as smoking, long-standing diabetes, dyslipidemia, or cocaine use.

CORONARY ARTERY DISEASE

Risk factors for coronary artery disease (CAD) in the childbearing age group include cigarette smoking, family history of premature CAD, an atherogenic lipid profile, diabetes mellitus, hypertension, preeclampsia, oral contraceptive use, and cocaine use.

These and other risk factors for CAD are discussed in the 2011 update to the American Heart Association guideline for the prevention of cardiovascular disease in women.

Pregnancy contributes to these risk factors by increasing total cholesterol, low-density lipoprotein, and triglycerides, and decreasing high-density lipoproteins.

Also, spontaneous coronary artery dissection and coronary spasm have been described more frequently as a cause for acute myocardial infarction in pregnant than in nonpregnant patients.

There are several case reports in the literature describing the management of delivery in women with coronary artery disease, ranging from spontaneous delivery with or without epidural analgesia to elective caesarean under combined spinal-epidural anaesthesia or elective caesarean under general anaesthesia.

MYOCARDIAL INFARCTION

Myocardial infarction was a leading cause of cardiac death in 2003-5; all the women who died had identifiable risk factors including obesity, older age and high parity, smoking, diabetes, pre-existing hypertension, and a family history.

Myocardial infarction complicating pregnancy is a rare occurrence, with an estimated incidence in the US of 1 in 10,000 pregnancies.

The risk of myocardial infarction is 3-4 fold higher in pregnancy when compared to nonpregnant reproductive age women, and the incidence is expected to rise owing to increasing maternal age.

A low threshold for diagnosis of myocardial infarction and acute coronary syndrome in women with risk factors is recommended and appropriate intervention in the form of coronary angiography, emergency coronary intervention, and thrombolysis should not be withheld in the pregnant or puerperal woman.

The diagnosis of myocardial infarction in pregnancy is established in the same way as in the nonpregnant state because clinical symptoms and investigations of infarction are not routinely affected by pregnancy.

Creatinine kinase and its MB fraction may be increased around the time of delivery.

Treatment is also generally the same in pregnancy with consideration of fetal effects.

Low-dose aspirin is considered safe during pregnancy; however, prolonged use of 100 mg aspirin can cause increased maternal bleeding complications and low birth weight.

Beta-blockers are the drug of choice in pregnancy due to their safety profile, while nitrates and calcium channel blockers should be used with caution to avoid maternal hypotension.

Thrombolytic therapy has limited data in pregnancy; no reports of teratogenic effects exist, but an increased risk of maternal hemorrhage exists.

The 2004 ACC/AHA guidelines consider pregnancy a relative contraindication to thrombolytic therapy.

Thrombolysis at the time of delivery carries a significant risk of haemorrhage and management therefore needs to be on an individual basis.

Coronary reperfusion by percutaneous transluminal coronary angioplasty or coronary bypass graft surgery has been reported with favorable outcomes.

The highest mortality in these cases has been in patients who have a myocardial infarction within the late third trimester.

This is likely due to the hemodynamic stress and cardiac decompensation that can occur in the peripartum period.

If possible, delivery has been suggested to be delayed for at least 2-3 weeks after an acute MI.

Management during labor and delivery should focus on minimizing cardiac workload during delivery.

Epidural anesthesia, medical management of hypertension, and possible invasive hemodynamic monitoring may be needed in labor.

Vaginal delivery is still reasonable unless other obstetrical indications exist, although an assisted vaginal delivery is preferred to avoid a prolonged second stage.

The need for anti-platelet medications (e.g. clopidogrel) would at present preclude the use of regional analgesia or anaesthesia.

SPECIFIC HIGH-RISK CONDITIONS

AORTIC DISSECTION

Aortic dissection is a particular risk in women with Marfan's syndrome; however, it can also occur in previously apparently normal women.

The risk is thought to be highest near full-term or the immediate post-partum period, in particular in the presence of systolic hypertension.

In the recent CEMACH report, an inappropriate emphasis on the treatment of diastolic hypertension led to failure to treat systolic hypertension in some of the women who died from aortic dissection.

In three out of the nine deaths from aortic dissection, there may also have been undiagnosed Marfan's syndrome.

The management of women with known Marfan's syndrome should include pre-pregnancy counselling if possible.

If the aortic root diameter is >4-4.5 cm, the risk of aortic dissection is greatly increased, so aortic root replacement should be offered before pregnancy.

ß-Blockers should be continued or started in pregnant patients with Marfan's syndrome who have aortic dilatation or hypertension as they have been found to reduce the rate of aortic dilatation.

Monitoring during pregnancy will normally include regular (e.g. every 4-8 weeks) transthoracic echocardiography to assess aortic root diameter.

The timing of delivery will be dependent on the root diameter and the rate of dilatation, and also any other complicating factors

The differential diagnosis of aortic dissection includes pulmonary embolism, pneumonia, pneumothorax, myocardial ischaemia, pericarditis, and musculoskeletal pain.

A recent case report demonstrates the difficulty of differentiating between some of these in the acute situation.

The occurrence of severe chest pain requiring opioid analgesia should always prompt investigation, including CT scan or transoesophageal echocardiogram where aortic dissection is suspected.

PULMONARY HYPERTENSION

Pulmonary arterial hypertension carries a very high risk during pregnancy (30-50% mortality).

If possible, this needs to be discussed pre-conception; if this has not been possible, it is appropriate in most cases for the question of termination to be raised and discussed with the mother, ideally by the multidisciplinary team who has carried out her risk assessment and who can advise on further management.

If the decision is made to continue with the pregnancy, efforts will be made to optimize her condition, usually including the use of a pulmonary arterial vasodilator such (e.g. sildenafil).

Owing to the increased risk of mortality at delivery, most units tend to opt for elective ceesarean section under a 'cardiac' general anaesthetic, as this allows control over ventilation, permits more invasive monitoring (e.g. transoesophageal echocardiography), and may lead to greater cardiovascular stability.

However, successful management using regional anaesthesia for caesarean section has also been described in pulmonary hypertension.

REFERENCES

− ACC/AHA guidelines for the management of patients with valvular heart disease. A report of the American College of Cardiology/American Heart Association. Task Force on Practice Guidelines (Committee on Management of Patients with Valvular Heart Disease). J Am Coll Cardiol. 1998; 32: 1486-588.

− Actis Dato GM, Cavaglia M, Aidala E, et al. Patent ductus arteriosus. Follow-up of 677 operated cases 40 years later. Minerva Cardioangiol. 1999; 47: 245-54.

− Actis Dato GM, Rinaudo P, Revelli A, et al. Atrial septal defect and pregnancy: a retrospective analysis of obstetrical outcome before and after surgical correction. Minerva Cardioangiol. 1998; 46: 63-8.

− ATS/ACCP Statement on cardiopulmonary exercise testing. Am J Respir Crit Care Med. 2003; 167: 211-77.

− Avila WS, Rossi EG, Ramires JA, et al. Pregnancy in patients with heart disease: experience with 1,000 cases. Clin Cardiol. 2003; 26: 135-42.

− Bates SM, Greer IA, Pabinger I, et al. Venous thromboembolism, thrombophilia, antithrombotic therapy and pregnancy: American College of Chest Physicians Evidence Based Clinical Practice Guidelines. Chest. 2008; 133: 844S.

− Beauchesne LM, Connolly HM, Ammash NM, et al. Coarctation of the aorta: outcome of pregnancy. J Am Coll Cardiol. 2001; 38: 1728-33.

− Bhargava B, Agarwal R, Yadav R, et al. Percutaneous balloon aortic valvuloplasty during pregnancy: use of the Inoue balloon and the physiologic antegrade approach. Cathet Cardiovasc Diagn. 1998; 45: 422-5.

– Bhatla N, Lal S, Behera G, et al. Cardiac disease in pregnancy. Int J Gynaecol Obstet. 2003; 82: 153-9.

– Bonow RO, Carabello BA, Chatterjee K et al. ACC/AHA 2006 Guidelines for the Management of Patients With Valvular Heart Disease. Circulation. 2006; 114: e84-e231.

– Borghi C, Esposti DD, Immordino V, et al. Relationship of systemic hemodynamics, left ventricular structure and function, and plasma natriuretic peptide concentrations during pregnancy complicated by preeclampsia. Am J Obstet Gynecol. 2000; 183: 140-7.

– Boyle RK. Anaesthesia in parturients with heart disease: a five year review in an Australian tertiary hospital. Int J Obstet Anesth. 2003; 12: 173-7.

– Bozkurt B, Villaneuva FS, Holubkov R, et al. Intravenous immune globulin in the therapy of peripartum cardiomyopathy. J Am Coll Cardiol. 1999; 34: 177-80.

– Boztosum B, Oleay A, Avei A, et al. Treatment of acute myocardial infarction in pregnancy with coronary artery balloon angioplasty and stenting: Use of tirofiban and clopidogrel. Int J Cardiol. 2008; 127: 413-6.

– Briggs GG, Freeman RK, Yaffe SJ. Drugs in Pregnancy and Lactation. 6th edition. Baltimore, MD: Lippincott Williams and Wilkins; 2002: 421, 1461.

– Brizzi P, Tonolo G, Esposito F, et al. Lipoprotein metabolism during normal pregnancy. Am J Obstet Gynecol. 1999; 181: 430-4.

– Campuzano K, Roque H, Bolnick A, et al. Bacterial endocarditis complicating pregnancy: case report and systematic review of the literature. Arch Gynecol Obstet. 2003; 268: 251-5.

– Caritis S, Sibai B, Hauth J, et al. Low-dose aspirin to prevent preeclampsia in women at high risk. National Institute of Child Health and Human Development Network of Maternal-Fetal Medicine Units. N Engl J Med. 1998; 338: 701-5.

– Chen FG, Koh KF, Chong YS. Cardiac arrest associated with sulprostone use during caesarean section. Anaesth Intensive Care. 1998; 26: 298-301.

– Cohen F, Garty M. Diuretics in pregnancy. In: Elkayam U, Gleicher N, editors. Cardiac Problems in Pregnancy. New York, NY: Wiley-Liss; 1998: 351-8.

– Colletti PM, Lee K. Cardiovascular imaging in the pregnant patient. In: Elkayam U, Gleicher N, editors. Cardiac Problems in Pregnancy. 3rd ed. New York: Wiley-Liss; 1998: 39-53.

– Cotrufo M, De Feo M, De Santo LS, et al. Risk of warfarin during pregnancy with mechanical valve prostheses. Obstet Gynecol. 2002; 99: 35-40.

– Dajani AS, Taubert KA, Wilson W, et al. Prevention of bacterial endocarditis. Recommendations by the American Heart Association. JAMA. 1997; 277: 1794-801.

– Daliento L, Somerville J, Presbitero P, et al. Eisenmenger syndrome. Factors relating to deterioration and death. Eur Heart J. 1998; 19: 1845-55.

– De Santo LS, Romano G, Della Corte A, et al. Mitral mechanical replacement in young rheumatic women: analysis of long-term survival, valve-related complications, and pregnancy outcomes over a 3707-patient-year follow-up. J Thorac Cardiovasc Surg. 2005; 130: 13-9.

– de Souza JA, Martinez EE Jr, Ambrose JA, et al. Percutaneous balloon mitral valvuloplasty in comparison with open mitral valve commissurotomy for mitral stenosis during pregnancy. J Am Coll Cardiol. 2001; 37: 900-3.

– Drenthen W, Pieper PG, Roos-Hesselink JW et al. Outcome of pregnancy in women with congenital heart disease: a literature review. J Am Coll Cardiol. 2007; 49: 2303.

– Drenthen W, Pieper PG, Roos-Hesselink JW et al. Pregnancy and delivery in women after Fontan palliation. Heart. 2006; 92: 1290-4.

– Drenthen W, Pieper PG, Roos-Hesselink JW, et al. Outcome of Pregnancy in woman with congenital heart disease. J Am Coll Cardiol. 2007; 49: 2303.

– Dua S, Maurtua MA, Cywinski JB. Anaesthetic management for emergency caesarean section in a patient with severe valvular disease and preeclampsia. Int J Obstet Anesth. 2006; 15: 250-3.

– Dwyer BK, Taylor L, Fuller A, et al. Percutaneous transluminal coronary angioplasty and stent placement in pregnancy. Obstet Gynecol. 2005; 106: 1162-4.

– Elkayam U, Akhter MW, Singh H, et al. Pregnancy-associated cardiomyopathy: clinical characteristics and a comparison between early and late presentation. Circulation. 2005; 111: 2050-5.

– Elkayam U, Dave R. Hypertrophic cardiomyopathy and pregnancy. In: Elkayam U, Gleicher N, editors. Cardiac Problems in Pregnancy. 3rd ed. New York: Wiley-Liss; 1998: 211-21.

– Elkayam U, Gleicher N. Cardiac evaluation during pregnancy. In: Elkayam U, Gleicher N, editors. Cardiac Problems in Pregnancy. 3rd ed. New York: Wiley-Liss; 1998: 39-53.

– Elkayam U, Tummala PP, Rao K, et al. Maternal and fetal outcomes of subsequent pregnancies in women with peripartum cardiomyopathy. N Engl J Med. 2001; 344: 1567-71.

– Elkayam U. Pregnancy and cardiovascular disease. In: Braunwald E, editor. Heart Disease: A Textbook of Cardiovascular Medicine. Philadelphia: WB Saunders; 2005: 1965-81.

– Evans PJ, Rajappan K, Stocks GM. Cardiorespiratory symptoms during pregnancy -- not always pulmonary embolism. Int J Obstet Anesth. 2006; 15: 320-4.

– Furman B, Shoham-Vardi I, Bashiri A, et al. Clinical significance and outcome of preterm prelabor rupture of membranes: population-based study. Eur J Obstet Gynecol Reprod Biol. 2000; 92: 209-16.

– Gil S, Atienzar C, Filella Y, et al. Anaesthetic management of acute myocardial infarction during labour. Int J Obstet Anesth. 2006; 15: 71-4.

– Gunderson EP, Lewis CE, Murtaugh MA, et al. Long-term plasma lipid changes associated with a first birth: the Coronary Artery Risk Development in Young Adults study. Am J Epidemiol. 2004; 159: 1028-39.

– Hameed A, Karaalp IS, Tummala PP, et al. The effect of valvular heart disease on maternal and fetal outcome of pregnancy. J Am Coll Cardiol. 2001; 37: 893-9.

– Hameed AB, Tummala PP, Goodwin TM, et al. Unstable angina during pregnancy in two patients with premature coronary atherosclerosis and aortic stenosis in association with familial hypercholesterolemia. Am J Obstet Gynecol. 2000; 182: 1152-5.

– Jamieson WR, Miller DC, Akins CW, et al. Pregnancy and bioprostheses: influence on structural valve deterioration. Ann Thorac Surg. Aug 1995; 60: S282-7.

– Kansaria JJ, Salvi VS. Eisenmenger syndrome in pregnancy. J Postgrad Med. 2000; 46: 101-3.

– Krishnamurthy M, Desai R, Patel H. Spontaneous coronary artery dissection in the postpartum period: association with antiphospholipid antibody. Heart. 2004; 90: e53.

– Kuczkowski KM, van Zundert A. Anesthesia for pregnant women with valvular heart disease: the state-of-the-art. J Anesth. 2007; 21: 252-7.

– Ladner HE, Danielsen B, Gilbert WM. Acute Myocardial Infarction in Preganncy and the Puerperium: A population based study. Am J Obstet Gynecol. 2005; 105: 480-4.

– Lao TT, Sermer M, Colman JM. Pregnancy after the Fontan procedure for tricuspid atresia. A case report. J Reprod Med. 1996; 41: 287-90.

– Lesniak-Sobelga A, Tracz W, KostKiewicz M, et al. Clinical and echocardiographic assessment of pregnant women with valvular heart diseases--maternal and fetal outcome. Int J Cardiol. 2004; 94: 15-23.

– Lewis G, editor. The Confidential Enquiry into Maternal and Child Health (CEMACH). Saving Mothers' Lives: reviewing maternal deaths to make motherhood safer 2003-2005. The Seventh Report on Confidential Enquiries into Maternal Deaths in the United Kingdom. London: CEMACH; 2007.

– Mason JW, O'Connell JB, Herskowitz A, et al. A clinical trial of immunosuppressive therapy for myocarditis. The Myocarditis Treatment Trial Investigators. N Engl J Med. 1995; 333: 269-75.

– Meijer JM, Pieper PG, Drenthen W, et al. Pregnancy, fertility, and recurrence risk in corrected tetralogy of Fallot. Heart. 2005; 91: 801-5.

- Mielniczuk LM, Williams K, Davis DR, et al. Frequency of peripartum cardiomyopathy. Am J Cardiol. 2006; 97: 1765-8.

- Mohler ER 3rd, Sorensen LC, Ghali JK, et al. Role of cytokines in the mechanism of action of amlodipine: the PRAISE Heart Failure Trial. Prospective Randomized Amlodipine Survival Evaluation. J Am Coll Cardiol. 1997; 30: 35-41.

- Mosca L, Benjamin EJ, Berra K, et al. Effectiveness-based guidelines for the prevention of cardiovascular disease in women--2011 update: a guideline from the american heart association. Circulation. 2011; 123: 1243-62.

- Nelson-Piercy C. Heart disease. In: Nelson-Piercy C, editor. Handbook of Obstetric Medicine, 2nd ed. Martin Dunitz: Taylor & Francis Group; 2002.

- Nieminen HP, Jokinen EV, Sairanen HI. Late results of pediatric cardiac surgery in Finland: a population-based study with 96% follow-up. Circulation. 2001; 104: 570-5.

- Nitsche JF, Phillips SD, Rose CH, et al. Pregnancy and delivery in patients with Fontan circulation. A case report and review of obstetric management. Obstet Gynocol Survey. 2009; 64: 607-14.

- North RA, Sadler L, Stewart AW, et al. Long-term survival and valve-related complications in young women with cardiac valve replacements. Circulation. 1999; 99: 2669-76.

- Packer M, Bristow MR, Cohn JN, et al. The effect of carvedilol on morbidity and mortality in patients with chronic heart failure. U.S. Carvedilol Heart Failure Study Group. N Engl J Med. 1996; 334: 1349-55.

- Parry AJ, Westaby S. Cardiopulmonary bypass during pregnancy. Ann Thorac Surg. 1996; 61: 1865-9.

– Paulson RJ, Boostanfar R, Saadat P, et al. Pregnancy in the sixth decade of life: obstetric outcomes in women of advanced reproductive age. JAMA. 2002; 288: 2320-3.

– Pearson GD, Veille JC, Rahimtoola S, et al. Peripartum cardiomyopathy: National Heart, Lung, and Blood Institute and Office of Rare Diseases (National Institutes of Health) workshop recommendations and review. JAMA. 2000; 283: 1183-8.

– Petanovic M, Zagar Z. The significance of asymptomatic bacteremia for the newborn. Acta Obstet Gynecol Scand. 2001; 80: 813-7.

– Plunkett MD, Bond LM, Geiss DM. Staged repair of acute type I aortic dissection and coarctation in pregnancy. Ann Thorac Surg. 2000; 69: 1945-7.

– Qasqas SA, McPherson C, Frishman WH, et al. Cardiovascular pharmacotherapeutic considerations during pregnancy and lactation. Cardiol Rev. 2004; 12: 201-21.

– Quinn J, Von Klemperer K, Brooks R, et al. Use of high intensity adjusted dose low moleclar weight heparin in women with mechanical heart valves during pregnancy: a single center experience. Haematologica. 2009; 94: 1608-12.

– Reimold SC, Rutherford JD. Clinical practice. Valvular heart disease in pregnancy. N Engl J Med. 2003; 349: 52-9.

– Romem A, Romem Y, Katz M, et al. Incidence and characteristics of maternal cardiac arrhythmias during labor. Am J Cardiol. 2004; 93: 931-3.

– Roth A, Elkayam U. Acute myocardial infarction and pregnancy. In: Elkayam U, Gleicher N, editors. Cardiac Problems in Pregnancy. 3rd ed. New York: Wiley-Liss; 1998: 121-30.

- Roth A, Elkayam U. Acute Myocardial Infarction Associated with Pregnancy. J Am Coll Cardiol. 2008; 52: 171-80.

- Sadler L, McCowen L, White H et al. Pregnancy outcomes and cardiac complication in women with mechanical, bioprosthetic and homograft valves. BJOG. 2000; 107: 245.

- Saidi AS, Bezold LI, Altman CA, et al. Outcome of pregnancy following intervention for coarctation of the aorta. Am J Cardiol. 1998; 82: 786-8.

- Salazar E, Espinola N, Roman L, et al. Effect of pregnancy on the duration of bovine pericardial bioprostheses. Am Heart J. 1999; 137: 714-20.

- Shapira Y, Sagie A, Battler. Low-molecular weight heparin for the treatment of patients with mechanical heart valves. Clin Cardiol. 2002; 25: 323.

- Silversides CK, Colman JM, Sermer M, et al. Cardiac risk in pregnant women with rheumatic mitral stenosis. Am J Cardiol. 2003; 91: 1382-5.

- Siu SC, Colman JM, Sorensen S, et al. Adverse neonatal and cardiac outcomes are more common in pregnant women with cardiac disease. Circulation. 2002; 105: 2179-84.

- Siu SC, Colman JM. Heart disease and pregnancy. Heart. 2001; 85: 710-5.

- Siu SC, Sermer M, Harrison DA, et al. Risk and predictors for pregnancy-related complications in women with heart disease. Circulation. 1997; 96: 2789-94.

- Smith RL, Young SJ, Greer IA. The Parturient with coronary heart disease. Int J Obstet Anesth. 2008; 17: 46-52.

− Soler-Soler J, Galve E. Worldwide perspective of valve disease. Heart. 2000; 83: 721-5.

− Somerville J. The Denolin Lecture: The woman with congenital heart disease. Eur Heart J. 1998; 19: 1766-75.

− Steer PJ, Gatzoulis MA, Baker P. Heart Disease and Pregnancy. London: RCOG Press; 2006.

− Steer PJ. Pregnancy and contraception. In: Gatzoulis MA, Swan L, Therrien J, Pantely GA, editors. Adult congenital heart disease: A practical guide. Oxford: BMJ Publishing, Blackwell Publishing; 2005: 16-35.

− Stout K. Pregnancy in women with congenital heart disease: the importance of evaluation and counselling. Heart. 2005; 91: 713-4.

− Stout KK, Otto CM. Pregnancy in women with valvular heart disease. Heart. 2007; 93: 552-8.

− Subtil D, Goeusse P, Puech F, et al. Aspirin (100 mg) used for prevention of pre-eclampsia in nulliparous women: the Essai Régional Aspirine Mère-Enfant study (Part 1). BJOG. 2003; 110: 475-84.

− Tamhane P, O'sullivan G, Reynolds F. Oxytocin in parturients with cardiac disease. Int J Obstet Anesth. 2006; 15: 332-3.

− Thaman R, Varnava A, Hamid MS, et al. Pregnancy related complications in women with hypertrophic cardiomyopathy. Heart. 2003; 89: 752-6.

− Therrien J, Marx GR, Gatzoulis MA. Late problems in tetralogy of Fallot--recognition, management, and prevention. Cardiol Clin. 2002; 20: 395-404.

− Thorne S, Deanfield J. Long-term outlook in treated congenital heart disease. Arch Dis Child. 1996; 75: 6-8.

– Tumelero RT, Duda NT, Tognon AP, et al. Percutaneous balloon aortic valvuloplasty in a pregnant adolescent. Arq Bras Cardiol. 2004; 82: 98-101, 94-7.

– Turker G, Gurbet A, Ayca Aksu H. Continuous spinal analgesia in parturients with severe heart disease. Int J Obstet Anesth. 2007; 16: 297-8.

– Uebing A, Steer PJ, Yentis SM, et al. Pregnancy and congenital heart disease. BMJ. 2006; 332: 401-6.

– Van Driel D, Wesseling J, Sauer PJ, et al. Teratogen update: fetal effects after, in utero exposure to coumarins, overview of cases, follow-up findings, and pathogenesis. Teratology. 2002; 66: 127-40.

– van Oppen AC, Stigter RH, Bruinse HW. Cardiac output in normal pregnancy: a critical review. Obstet Gynecol. 1996; 87: 310-8.

– Veldtman GR, Connolly HM, Grogan M, et al. Outcomes of pregnancy in women with tetralogy of Fallot. J Am Coll Cardiol. 2004; 44: 174-80.

– Vitale N, DeFeo M, DeSanto LS. Dose-dependent fetal complications of warfarin in pregnant women with mechanical heart valves. J Am Coll Cardiol. 1999; 1637-41.

– Walker F. Pregnancy and teh various forms of the Fontan circulation. Heart. 2007; 93: 152-54.

– Warnes CA, Elkayam U. Congenital heart disease in pregnancy. In: Elkayam U, Gleicher N, editors. Cardiac Problems in Pregnancy. 3rd ed. New York, NY: Wiley-Liss; 1998: 39-55.

– Weiss BM, Hess O. Perioperative cardiovascular evaluation for noncardiac surgery: congenital heart diseases and heart diseases in pregnancy deserve better guidelines. Circulation. 1997; 95: 530-1.

– Weiss BM, Hess OM. Pulmonary vascular disease and pregnancy: current controversies, management strategies, and perspectives. Eur Heart J. 2000; 21: 104-15.

– Weiss BM, von Segesser LK, Alon E, et al. Outcome of cardiovascular surgery and pregnancy: a systematic review of the period 1984-1996. Am J Obstet Gynecol. 1998; 179: 1643-53.

– Whitehead SJ, Berg CJ, Chang J. Pregnancy-related mortality due to cardiomyopathy: United States, 1991-1997. Obstet Gynecol. 2003; 102: 1326-31.

– Witlin AG, Mabie WC, Sibai BM. Peripartum cardiomyopathy: an ominous diagnosis. Am J Obstet Gynecol. 1997; 176: 182-8.

– Yap SC, Drenthen W, Pieper PG, et al. Risk of complications during pregnancy in women with congenital aortic stenosis. Inter J of Card. 2008; 126: 240-6.